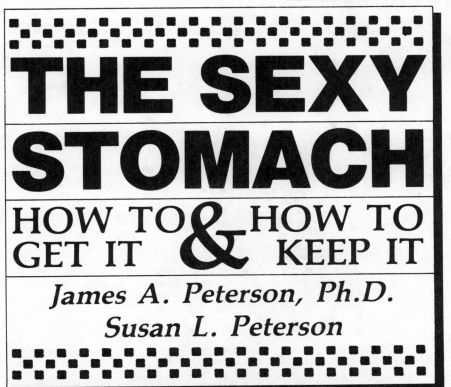

THE SEXY STOMACH

HOW TO GET IT & HOW TO KEEP IT

James A. Peterson, Ph.D.
Susan L. Peterson

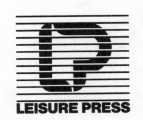

LEISURE PRESS

NEW YORK

A publication of
Leisure Press.
597 Fifth Avenue; New York, N.Y. 10017

Library of Congress Catalog Card Number: 82-83928

ISBN: 0-88011-096-1

Cover and book design: Brian Groppe
Cover photographs: David Madison
Text photographs: David Madison
Typesetting: The Graphics Connection; Oakland, California

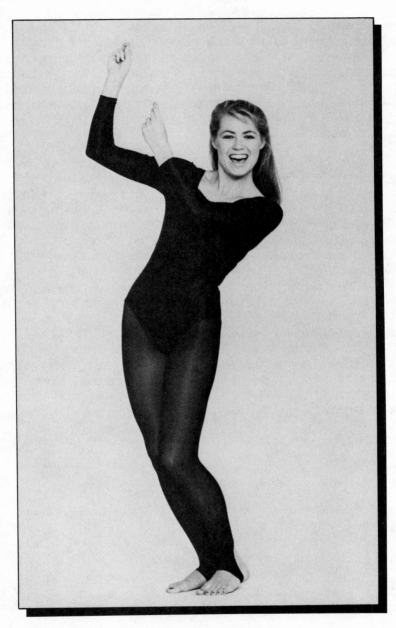

Your sexy stomach is just weeks away!

Pity the poor stomach. On the one hand, we ask it to serve a vital life sustaining function as a holding and processing tank for the food we eat; while on the other hand, we'd just as soon see our stomachs keep a low profile. They're constantly reminding us that we ate the wrong thing or too much of the right thing. Somewhat not surprisingly, stomachs come in all sizes: fat ones, thin ones, soft ones, semi-soft ones, hard ones, and so on. Obviously, you've decided that yours is somewhat less than as sexy as you'd like it to be since you purchased this book on rehabilitating stomach muscles.

Before you read too much further, however, we feel that it is only fair to warn you that you're facing a good news - bad news situation. The good news is that almost anyone can develop a sexy stomach. The bad news is that it requires work . . . and patience. There is no magic pill that will enable you to acquire a sexy stomach overnight, no Polybetzian elixir that will give you the will power to do what is necessary to whip your tummy into shape. All anyone can do for you is to give you the information on how to develop a sexy stomach. What you do with that information is up to you.

The exercises in this book—when combined with sensible eating habits—will develop your stomach to a degree perhaps beyond your wildest imagination. The flat, firm, sexy stomach you've always wanted is yours for the asking if you're willing to work for it. No one else can perform the exercises for you. You must do them . . . correctly, regularly and diligently. If you compromise the proper way of doing the exercises, you'll compromise your goal of having a sexy stomach.

Remember, sexy is in. Think sexy. Your sexy stomach is just weeks away.

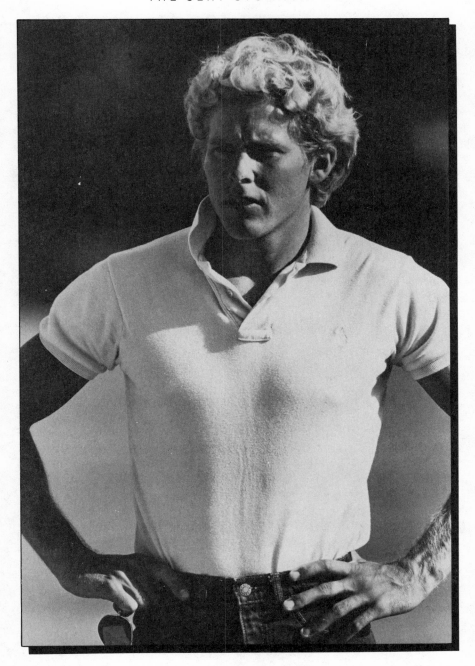

A sexy stomach can have a positive effect on both your physical health and mental well-being.

WHAT IS A SEXY STOMACH?

Sexy stomachs have several characteristics. They're firm and hard. They usually belong to *other* people. They allow their owners (of the sexy stomach) to wear the clothes they want without regard to how well those clothes can hide protruding bulges. They're the envy of all the owners' friends . . . and some of the owners' enemies as well. If you own one, it's usually worth a kind word or two from your family physician during your annual physical. But above all, a sexy stomach will contribute to your sense of physical and mental well-being.

Beauty, as the old adage goes, is in the eye of the beholder. If you think your stomach is sexy, then it's sexy. If you feel good about yourself, that's super. That's also what this book is all about—feeling good and looking terrific.

You may be wondering if it is necessary for you to look like Candice Bergen or Tom Sellick in order for you to have a sexy stomach. Emphatically no! Sexy stomachs are attainable by everyone—short people, tall people, brunettes, blondes, red heads, older adults, teenagers, you, us . . . literally everyone.

You know you don't have a sexy stomach when:

...You ask someone to sit on your lap and she asks 'which lap'?

...Your 18 hour girdle lasts 15 minutes.

...Someone must tell you when your shoes are not tied.

...Your bicycle salesman recommends a pizza plate for a seat.

WHY HAVE A SEXY STOMACH?

No one wants to be the brunt of a joke, even a funny one. But having a sexy stomach will do more for you than keep your tummy from being the subject of a personalized joke. A sexy stomach can have a positive effect on both your physical health and mental well-being.

The latest government health figures suggest that more than 30,000,000 Americans suffer from some degree of painful discomfort to their lower backs. The primary reason for this epidemic of pain is a lack of abdominal fitness by those who suffer back pain. Their unfit abdominal muscles protrude forward causing their back muscles to literally be pulled forward. In turn, this pulling on their back muscles causes a tightening in their lower back and places a considerable amount of stress on the nerve endings in that area of the spine. Viola, low back pain appears. Fortunately for suffers of low back pain, the reverse is also true. When your stomach muscles are tightened up, the level of support they provide to your stomach and other internal organs is increased. There is then a corresponding reduction in the amount of pulling tension on your lower back muscles. In turn, the stress on your spine and lower back is dissipated. Viola, the pain goes away. Is this simple explanation for back pain too good to be believed? Perhaps. Does it actually happen this way? Most definitely, yes.

The other basis for wanting to have a sexy stomach—and certainly as important as the physical reasons—is your mental well-being. It is very important for you to feel good about yourself. Let's face it, ours is basically a thin-is-in oriented society. Both the visual and print media—television, movies, magazines, newspapers, etc.—hammer that point incessantly at the public. Thin is **THE** look. Thin people are portrayed as glamorous, sociable, well-liked, intelligent, contemporary, opportunistic . . . in a word, successful.

As a result, it's only human nature for everyone to want to do whatever is necessary to be successful. To be sure, there are a limited number of people who've made "it" without a sexy stomach, but such cases are few and far between. Surely, they were successful in spite of their obvious lack of possessing a sexy stomach. If yours isn't what you feel it should be (signs of creeping obesity? a lateral love handle transplant?), perhaps, you reason, others will notice this deficiency in your personal commitment to success. Up goes you anxiety level, down goes your self-esteem. The potential consequences: problems with your social life; difficulties in your business relationships; uncertainties about your capabilities. Not good for your mental health. The suggested remedy—develop a sexy stomach.

THE PROGRAM

OK! OK! So we convinced you. Now what? You've already taken the critical first step—you've recognized the need to shape up your stomach. You've also taken the logical second step by obtaining accurate advice (the steps, exercises and programs described in this book) on how to accomplish your goal of overhauling your stomach muscles.

The next step is to identify what exercises to do and "put on your exercising shoes to beat the flabby tummy blues". Before you get started, however, (the exercises are described and illustrated in the next section of this book) we'd like to provide you with a few basic guidelines to follow in order to insure that your program will give you the greatest possible results, in the least amount of required time and in the safest possible manner.

GUIDELINES

1 Before beginning any exercise program, you should have a medical examination by a physician. Be sure to inform your physician of your intention to exercise. If an injury occurs or you become ill during your exercise program, consult your physician before continuing.

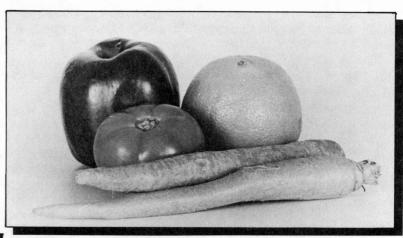

In order to truly develop a sexy stomach, you must combine your exercise program with sensible eating habits.

2 In order for you to truly develop a sexy stomach, you must combine your exercise program with sensible eating habits. It would be foolish to believe, for example, that anyone who excessively abused his or her body nutritionally could firm up his or her stomach muscles to the maximal desired level. You have to face it—certain foods when eaten in excess will prevent you from attaining a sexy stomach. An excellent source book on the subject of nutrition is *Jane Brody's Nutrition Book.*

3 The time of day to exercise is an individual matter. However, it would be wise for you to wait at least an hour after eating before exercising.

4 What you wear, where you exercise, whether you exercise with another person or alone are all personal decisions. It is in your best interest to make them prior to starting your exercise program if possible.

5 If you are relatively unaccustomed to strenuous exercise, you should start gradually by performing Level I (beginning) exercises. Your basic program should include at a minimum at least eight exercises at each level of intensity (I, II, III). We recommend that when you are initially performing the exercises at a particular intensity level, you do 6-8 repetitions of each exercise. Once you successfully complete 10-12 repetitions of most exercises at Level I, you can move up to Level II, or from Level II to Level III if you can comfortably do 10-12 repetitions of most of the Level II exercises.

6 Try to exercise at least 4-5 times a week. If you exercise regularly, you should see substantial improvement within a month. Remember, the more you exercise, the quicker the improvement will be. Be patient however. You didn't get out of shape overnight and you won't get into shape overnight. (Remember, the more you exercise, the quicker the improvement will be.)

7 You will achieve better results from these exercises if you perform them slowly and smoothly. Fast, jerky movements are ballistic in nature. Such movements are counterproductive to your goal of achieving a sexy stomach. When you exercise ballistically, your muscles are not required to do work throughout their full range of motion for each exercise. Literally, in this instance, you're merely throwing your body, not exercising it. When you perform exercises, in a fast, jerky manner, you're also subjecting yourself to an increased chance of being injured.

8 It is very important for your stomach muscles that you breathe normally and freely while exercising. You should never hold your breath while exercising.

9 Be careful not to arch your back (hyperextend) while performing those exercises which involve your lower back. If at all possible, always try to keep your lower back in contact with the floor.

10 While reading the directions for performing each exercise, be sure to pay special attention to the *Notes* written for certain exercises. All directions should be followed closely so that you perform every exercise correctly. Remember, if you compromise the way an exercise should be done, you compromise the results that you can achieve.

11 Your exercise program should include both warm-up and warm-down exercises, in addition to the stomach exercises.

12 Under normal circumstances, your exercise routine should take at least 15-20 minutes including warm-ups and warm-downs. Remember, don't be in a hurry while exercising your stomach muscles. You must perform the exercises properly if your program is to be both effective and safe.

13 Although exercising should not be painful, you may experience sore stomach muscles the first few days of your program. Do not quit exercising. Continue, but at a slower pace; use fewer repetitions, at a different level, etc. Under no circumstances, however, should you eliminate warm-ups and warm-downs from your workout. They're important. Do them every workout. A warm bath or shower may also be helpful. Keep in mind that although it may seem like a lifetime, muscle soreness will only last for a few days. If for some reason it lasts longer, either your program is much too arduous or you may have a medical problem which requires attention. Usually, it's your program. In that instance, you'll have to adjust it accordingly.

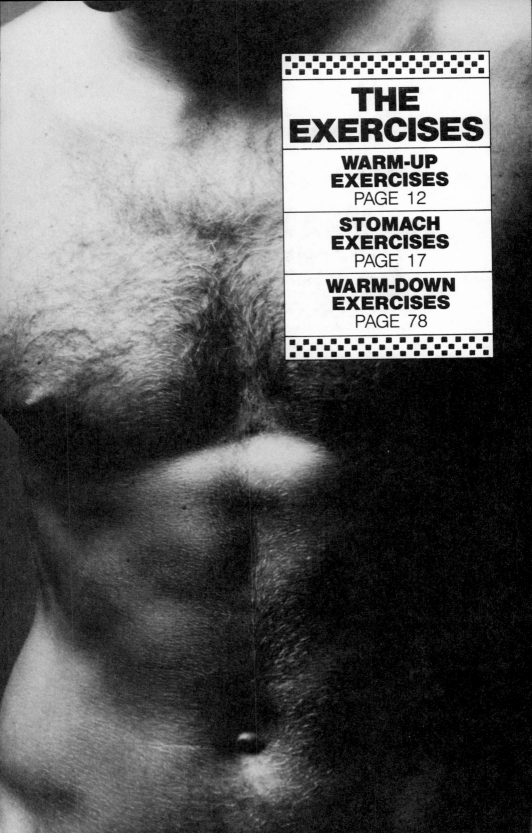

THE EXERCISES

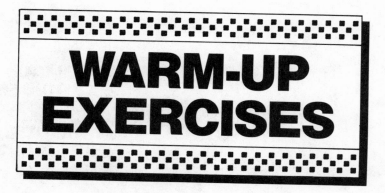

Warm-up exercises are intended to increase your circulation and raise the temperature in your muscles. They should be performed at the beginning of every exercise workout to prepare your body for strenuous activity. The primary objective of warm-ups is to prevent injury. All of the suggested exercises should be performed slowly and smoothly. Do not bounce or jerk while exercising. The amount of time you should spend on warm-ups is up to you. We recommend, however, that you devote at least 5 minutes to the warm-up portion of your routine.*

*These warm-ups are designed to begin from a seated or floor position so that less strain is put on your lower back. Since millions of people suffer from back problems, it is important that your back be protected as much as possible during the execution of every exercise.

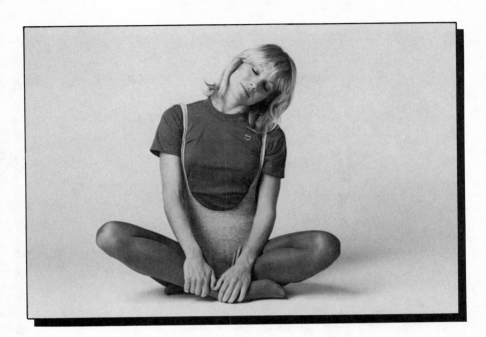

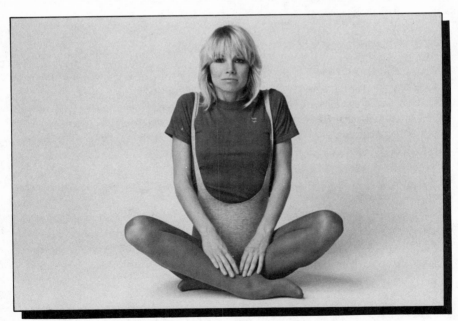

1 Sit in a comfortable position, do several head circles and shoulder shrugs.

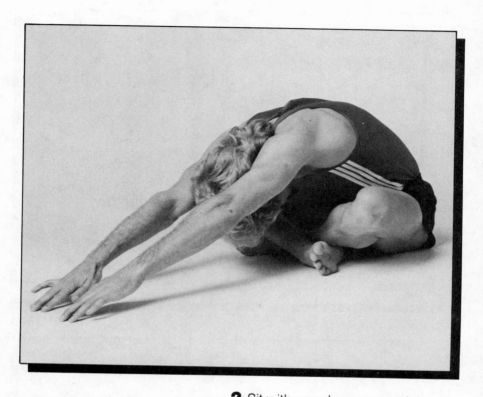

2 Sit with your legs crossed, bend forward at your trunk and reach along the floor with your fingertips for six counts. Slowly curl back up returning to a straight sitting position—dragging your hands along the floor towards you until you are sitting up again. Sit tall, take a deep breath, exhale and repeat the stretch slowly.

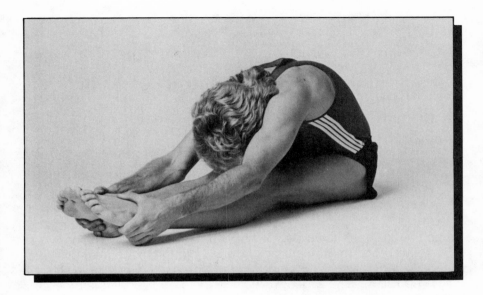

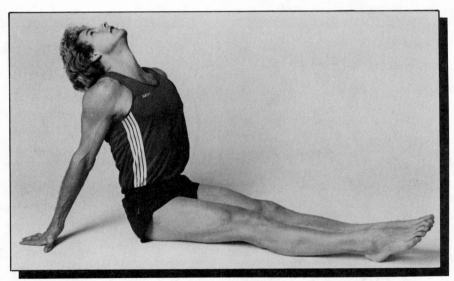

3 Sit with your legs extended, slowly bend forward and reach both of your hands toward your ankles, and hold for six counts. Slowly return to a straight sitting position (curling back upward). Place your hands on the floor behind you, look to the ceiling behind you while arching your back *very slightly* and hold for six counts. Return to a straight sitting position, take a deep breath, exhale and repeat the stretch.

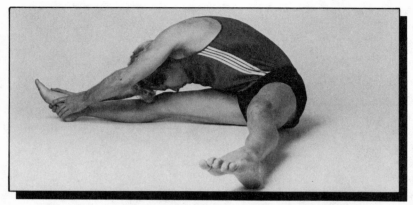

4 Sit with your legs apart, turn and reach your hands towards your right ankle and hold for six counts. Turn and reach to the center floor and hold for six counts; turn and reach toward your left ankle and hold for six counts. Return to a straight sitting position, take a deep breath, exhale and repeat, left, center, right, etc.

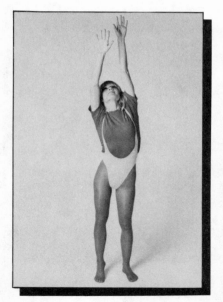

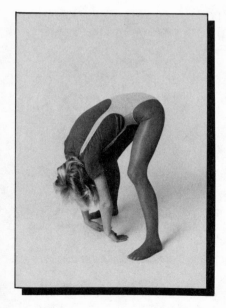

5 Stand with your legs slightly apart, look to the ceiling and reach both hands upwards six counts. Slowly bend at your waist and relax over for six counts (do not bounce, and keep your knees slightly bent). Curl up slowly for six counts to a standing position, and repeat reaching, etc.

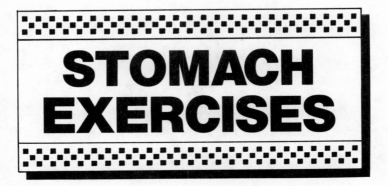

These exercises are divided into three groups. Level I exercises are designed for those individuals who are unaccustomed to strenuous exercise involving the abdominal muscles. Level II exercises are slightly more difficult than Level I exercises and should be performed by those individuals with an intermediate level of abdominal fitness. The most strenuous level of exercises is Level III—the level for advanced performers.

LEVEL I:
THE BEGINNER

ISOMETRIC
CONTRACTION

Sit or stand with good posture and pull in your stomach. Hold for 6-10 seconds; relax and repeat. Do not hold your breath! In fact, count or speak out loud to help prevent yourself from holding your breath. You can assist this action by placing your hands on your lower stomach and pushing down gently while you contract the muscles. *Note:* This contraction may also be done while moving around; e.g., walking, working, doing household chores, etc.

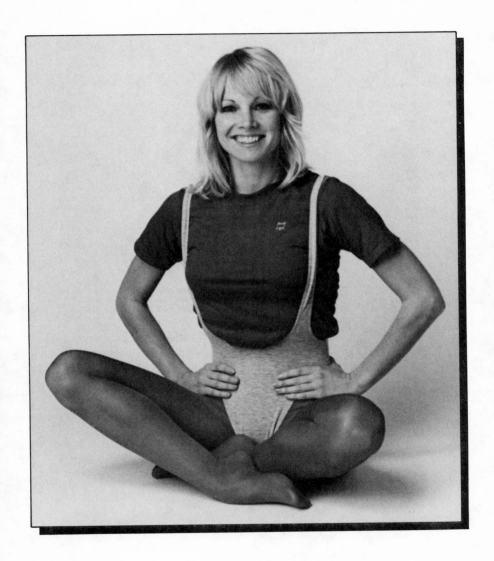

BACK PRESS

Assume the supine position (on your back) with your knees bent and your arms out at your shoulders. Pull in your stomach and press your lower back to the floor. Hold for 6-10 seconds. Relax and repeat.

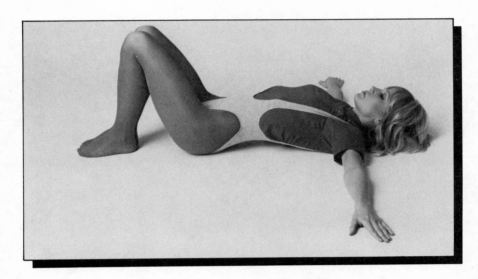

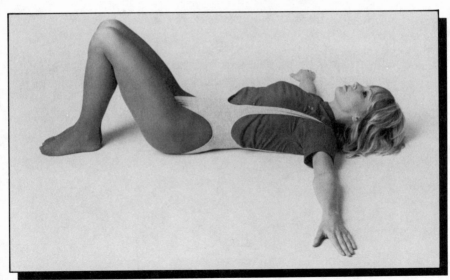

SINGLE LEG LIFTS

Assume a supine position (on your back) with your arms out at your shoulders. Bring your right knee to your chest, extend your leg up toward the ceiling (toes pointed), return it to your chest, and then to the floor. Repeat with your left leg, right, left, etc. in a rapid succession.

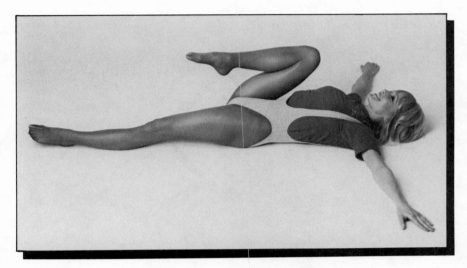

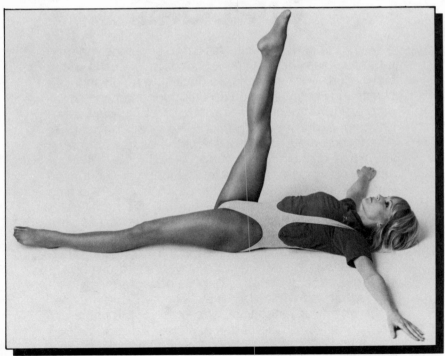

CURL-UPS

Assume a supine position with your knees bent, and your hands on your shoulders. Slowly curl your head forward (tucking your chin to your chest) and continue to curl up until your head and shoulders are off the floor (only about 12"-15"), pause and slowly uncurl down to the floor. Relax and repeat. Be sure to breathe freely throughout the exercise. *Note:* If you have difficulty performing the exercise with your hands resting on your shoulders, extend your hands forward and reach toward your knees while you are curling up. If you still cannot curl-up, do only the negative or downward portion of the exercise. From a seated position, just curl downward to the floor. Relax and then by using your hands, push yourself up off the floor to return to a seated position. Then, lower yourself down again. The advantage of performing these downward-only curl-ups is that you work (stress) exactly the same muscles in the downward (negative) phase as you do in the upward (positive) phase of this exercise. As soon as you are able, you should perform the curl-up in a normal fashion (e.g., do both the upward and the downward movements).

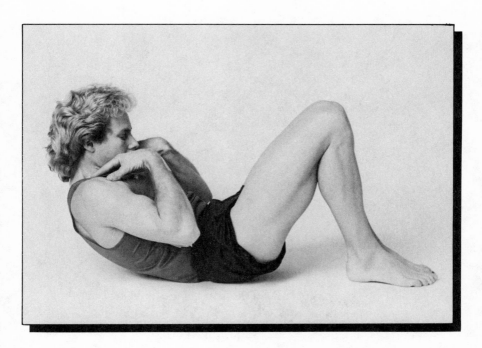

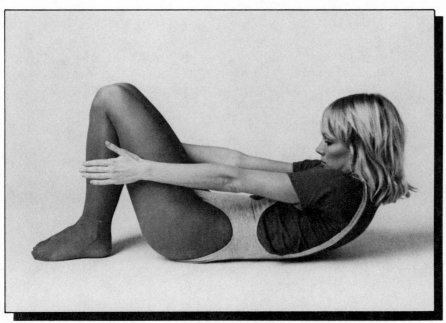

TRUNK TWIST

Sit with your legs together, toes pointed and hands on your shoulders. Twist your trunk to the left, and continue twisting for four counts while you look over your left shoulder. Repeat to your right, left, right, etc. *Note:* Do not let your hips turn while you do the exercise. You are in a seated rather than a standing position to stabilize your hips so they cannot assist with the twisting action of your trunk.

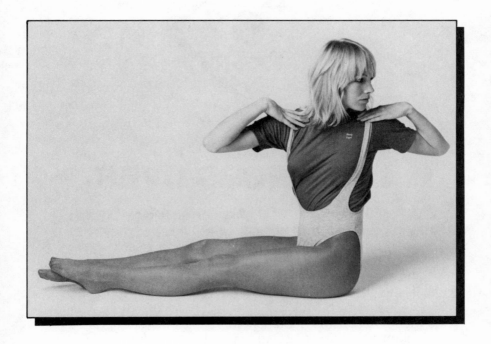

LEG CROSS-OVER

Assume a supine position with your arms held out at your shoulders. Slowly raise your right leg up (toes pointed) and lower it across your body toward your left hand. If this is too difficult, touch the floor at your waist level or above. Slowly return your leg to a straight up position and lower it to the floor. Repeat with your left leg, right, left, etc. *Note:* Keep your back, head, and shoulders in contact with the floor as much as possible during the exercise.

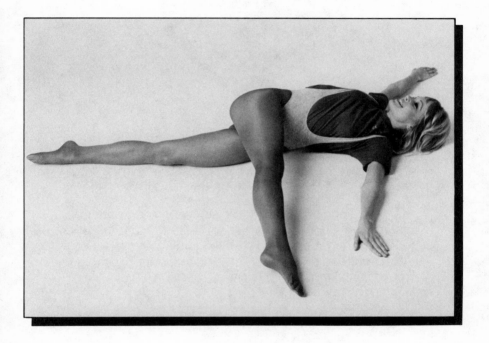

SEATED ELBOW-KNEE TOUCH

Sit with your legs apart, toes pointed and hands on your shoulders. Twist left and touch your right elbow to your left thigh (near the knee). Twist right and touch your left elbow to your right thigh. Repeat left, right, left, etc. in succession.

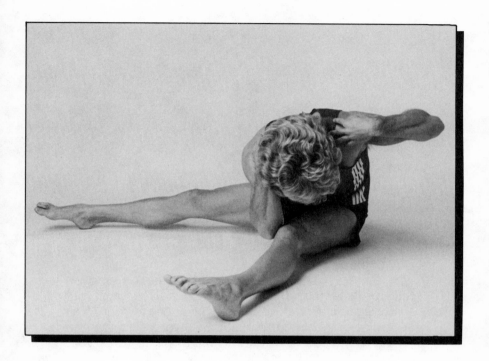

HIP LIFT

Assume a supine position with your knees bent, your feet flat on the floor, and your arms held out at your sides. Lift your knees to your chest and raise your hips off the floor. Lower your hips and repeat in succession. *Note:* If this exercise hurts your lower back or tailbone, put a towel under your hips.

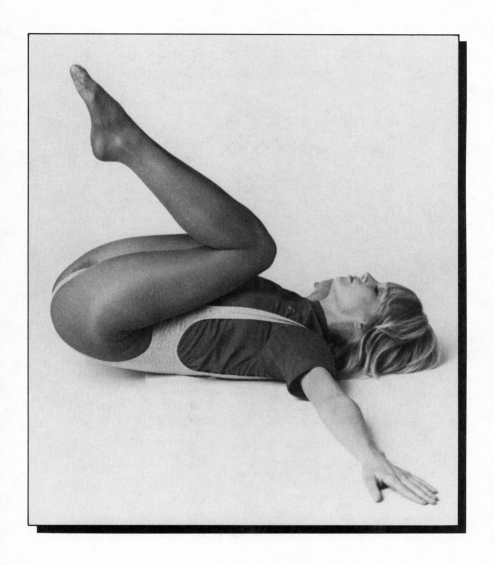

CAT STRETCH

On your hands and knees with your back straight, tuck your chin to your chest, and raise your back up as you pull in your stomach muscles (arch your back like a cat when it stretches). Relax and repeat. *Note:* Do not let your back sag at anytime during the exercise.

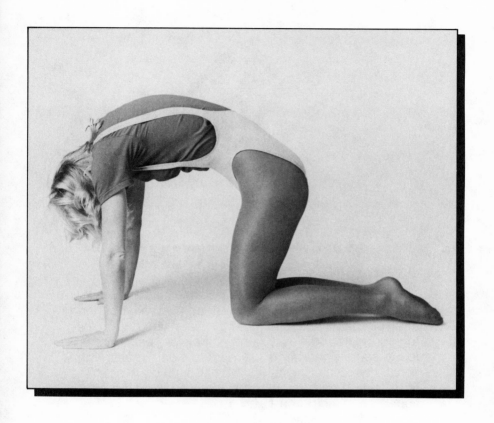

SIDE BENDING

Stand with your feet shoulder width apart, with your arms extended up over your head and your hands grasped together. Keep your arms close to your head and slowly bend to the side, pause, return to the center, and bend to the other side. Repeat right, center, left, center, right, etc. *Note:* Keep your hips stable and forward throughout the bend. You should not turn your hips to help you bend.

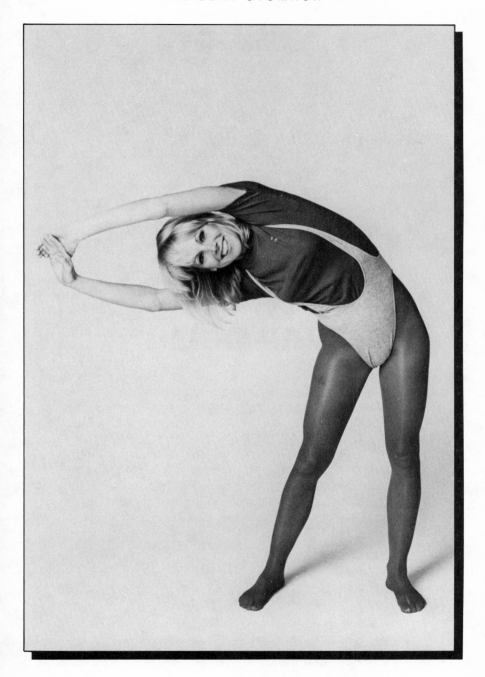

LEVEL II:
INTERMEDIATE

HIP ROLL

Assume a supine position with your arms held out at your shoulders. Bring both your knees in tight to your chest and slowly roll to your left side with your knees pointed up toward your elbow (hold you knees 1"-2" off the floor; don't let them touch the floor). Return to the center, roll to your right side, return to the center, and return both your legs to the floor to a full reclining position. Repeat left, center, right, center, floor, etc. *Note:* keep your head, shoulders and upper back on the floor as much as possible.

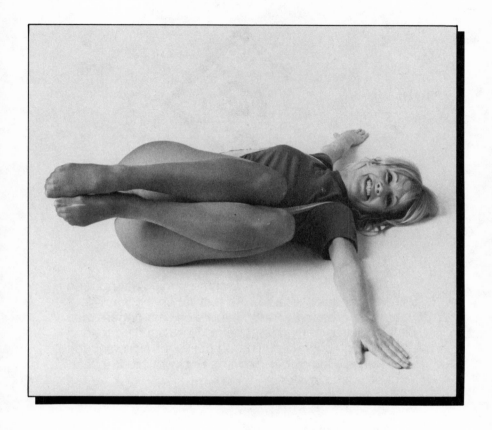

SIT-UPS

Assume a supine position with your knees bent and your feet flat on the floor. Your hands may rest on your shoulders or your fingers may be interlocked behind your head. Slowly curl your head toward and continue curling up until your elbows touch your knees. Return by uncurling backward to the floor. Repeat in succession.

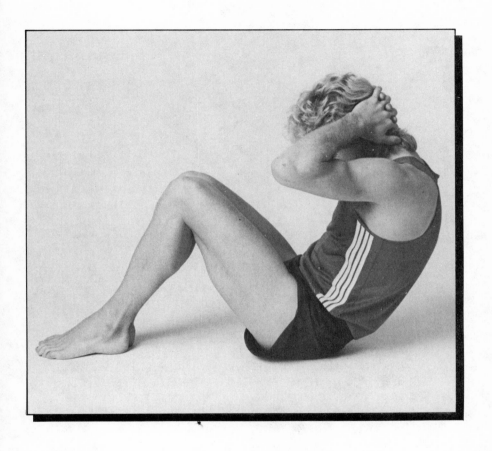

SIDE LYING DOUBLE LEG LIFT

Lie on your side with your legs extended one on top of the other, and your feet pointed up toward your shins (your ankles flexed toward you). Slowly raise both your legs off the floor and hold. Slowly lower your legs to the floor. Relax and repeat. Repeat the entire exercise on the opposite side of your body. *Note:* Be sure to keep your body in a straight line (you may help support yourself with your hands). Do not roll forward or backward.

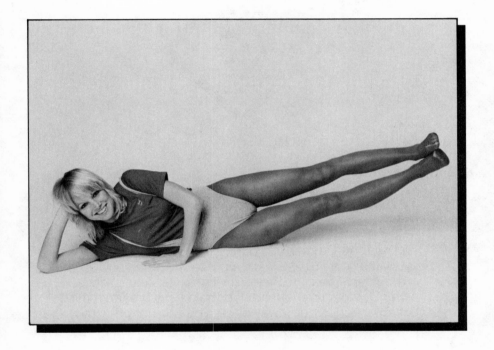

LEG CRISS-CROSS

Assume a supine position and support yourself on your elbows. Lift both your legs up off the floor (10″-12″) with your toes pointed and criss cross your legs at the thighs six times. Relax and repeat. *Note:* Do not arch your back or hold your breath. If this exercise hurts your lower back, you are not physically ready to perform it.

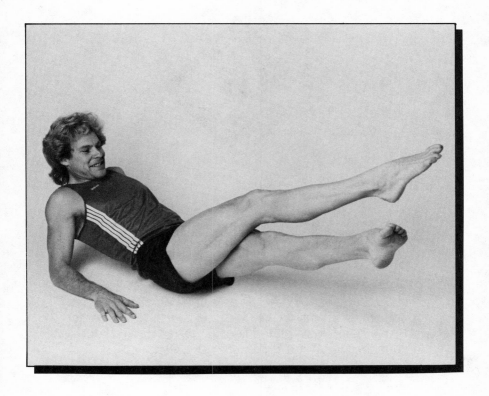

SIT-UP AND TWIST

Assume a supine position with your knees bent, your feet flat on the floor and your hands on your shoulders. Sit up and vigorously twist your trunk to the left as far as possible, return to the center and lay back down on the floor. Then, sit up and repeat in succession to the right, left, right, etc.

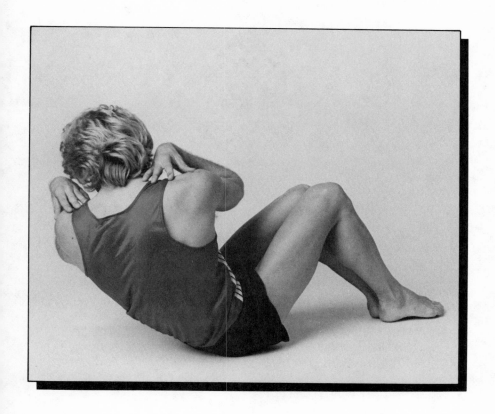

V-SIT

Sit with your arms held out at your shoulders. Lean backward and bring both your knees to your chest, get your balance, then quickly extend both legs straight up and forward to a V-sit position. Hold for 4-6 seconds. Relax and repeat. Breathe normally throughout the exercise.

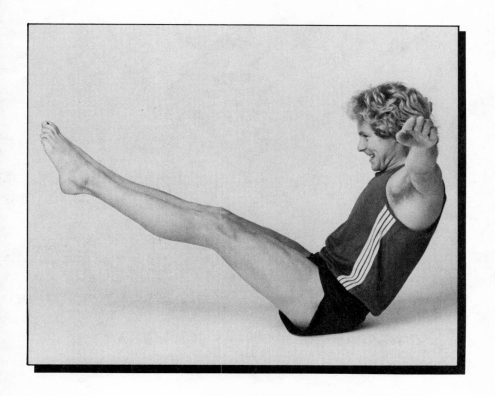

BICYCLE

Assume a supine position and support yourself on your elbows. Lift both your legs up off the floor (only 12"-15") and slowly move your legs in a bicycle pedaling fashion six times. Relax and repeat. *Note:* Bend your knees slightly as you pedal to keep the action horizontal. Do not arch your lower back.

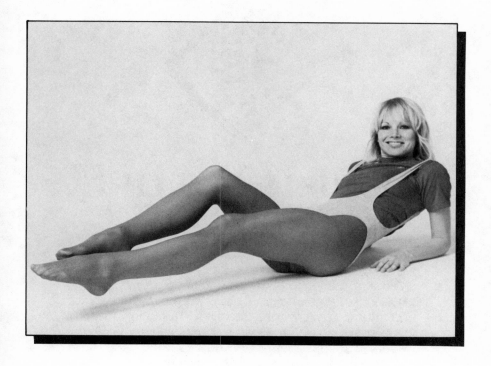

DOUBLE LEG LIFT EXTENSION

Assume a supine position with your legs extended and your arms held out at your shoulders. Bend both knees in toward your chest and extend both legs straight up toward the ceiling. Pause and return to a bent knee position. Then quickly extend your legs forward to the floor (the starting position). Repeat in succession. *Note:* Keep your hips and lower back on the floor as much as possible.

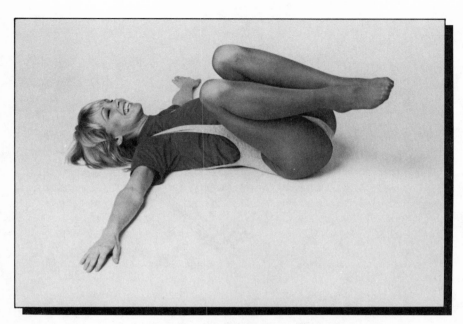

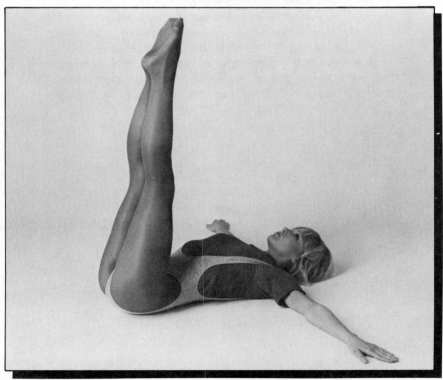

SIDE BICYCLE

In the same position as the bicycle exercise, roll onto your right hip. Keeping your head and shoulders facing forward, bicycle pedal to the right six times; roll onto your left hip and repeat. Relax and repeat right, left, right, left, etc. in succession.

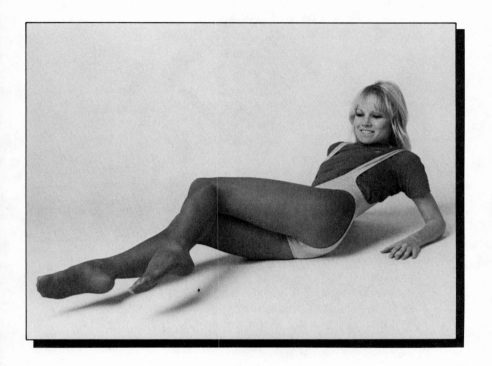

SIT-UP HEAD-KNEE TOUCH

Assume a supine position with your legs apart, your knees slightly bent and your arms extended overhead. Sit up to reach and touch both hands to your left ankle, reach to the center and touch the floor, reach and touch your right ankle, and then reassume a supine position on the floor. Repeat in succession left, center, right, etc.

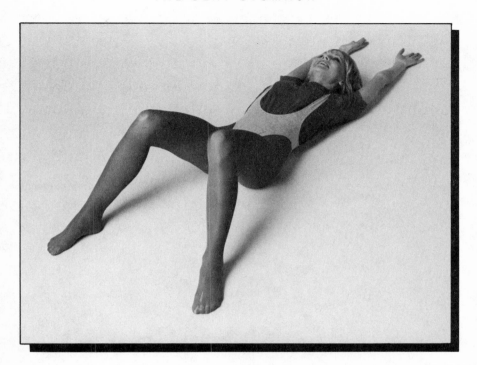

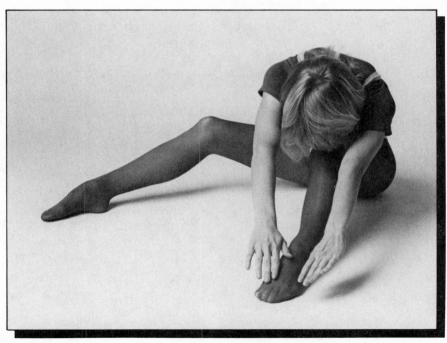

SIT-UP KNEE-GRASP

Assume a supine position with your knees bent and your hands on your shoulders. Sit-up and grasp your right knee with both hands touching your head to your knee. Hold, return to the supine position on the floor. Repeat sit-up and grasp your left knee, then your right, your left, etc., in succession.

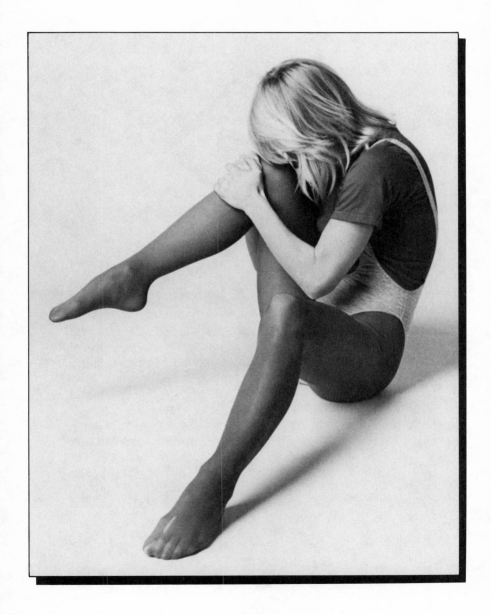

DOUBLE LEG LIFT

Assume a supine position and support yourself on your elbows. Keep your lower back in contact with the floor as much as possible. Bend both your knees in close to your chest, pause, then extend both legs to the front 12″-15″ off the floor, and slowly lower your legs to the floor. Relax and repeat. *Note:* Do not arch your lower back. Remember to breathe normally throughout the exercise. This exercise is not performed in the "traditional" supine position because too many people arch their back. If you find that you still arch your back in the elbow support position, do not perform this exercise. Properly and safely performed, it should not cause discomfort to your back.

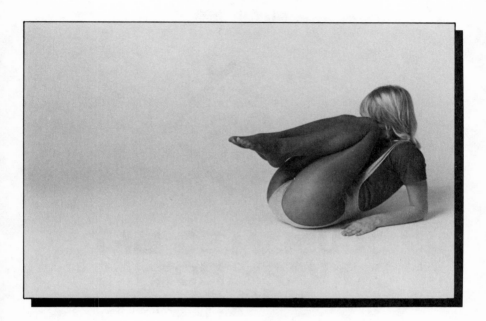

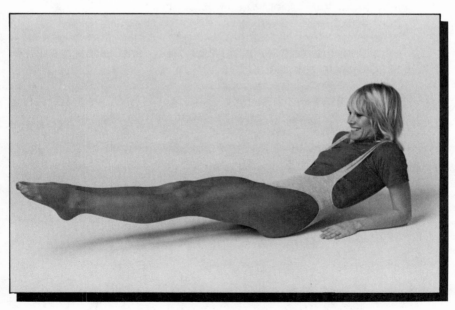

LEVEL III: ADVANCED

DOUBLE LEG LIFT VARIATION

Use the same starting position as for the double leg lift. Bring both your knees to your chest, extend your legs forward (still only 12″-15″ off the floor), separate them, bring them back together, and lower them slowly to the floor. Relax and repeat the sequence to a count of five.

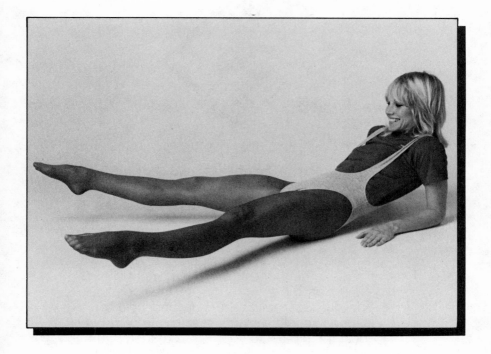

ADVANCED HIP ROLL

Assume a supine position with your arms out at your shoulders. Bring both your knees in tight to your chest, roll to your right side and lower your knees to the floor (1 "-2 " off the floor). Quickly extend your legs out to the side and hold for 4-6 seconds. Bend your knees and return to the center position. Repeat the hip roll to your left side; then return to the center and then to the floor or starting (supine) position. Relax and repeat sequence. *Note:* Keep your head, shoulders, and upper back on the floor as much as possible. Do not arch your back as you extend and hold your legs out to the side.

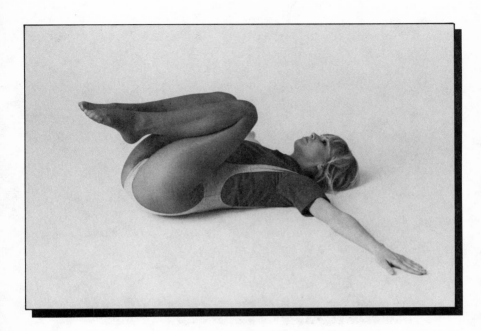

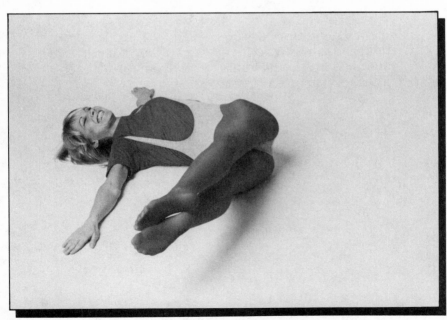

ADVANCED SIT-UP

Perform a Level II sit-up (#12) but vary your arm position as follows: either fold your arms across your chest while doing the sit-up or hold your arms up overhead at a level even with your ears throughout the sit-up.

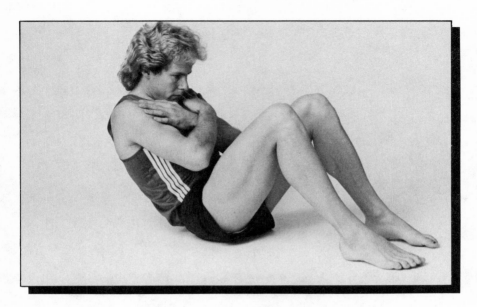

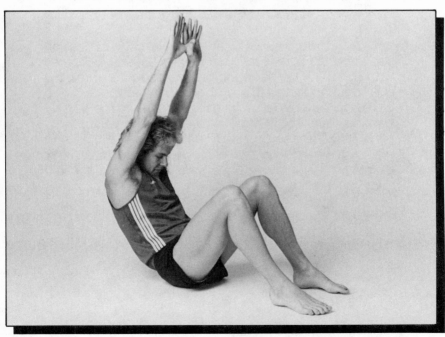

ADVANCED BICYCLE SEQUENCE

Assume a supine position and support yourself on your elbows. Lift both your legs up 12″-15″ off the floor and bicycle pedal six times; roll over onto your right hip and pedal six times; return to the center and pedal six times; and return to the starting position. This action involves continuous movement with no resting between the different positions. Relax and repeat to the center, right, center, left, center, etc. *Note:* Do not hold your breath while pedaling. Also, do not arch your lower back!

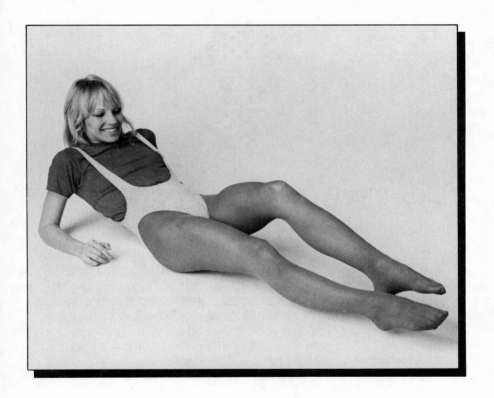

TRUNK TWISTING SIT-UPS

Sit with your knees bent, your feet flat on the floor and your hands on your shoulders. Turn to your left as far as possible and slowly curl backwards toward the floor (do not touch the floor); pause and remain twisted as you slowly curl up to a sitting position. Quickly turn to your right and repeat the sit-up. Repeat in succession to the left, right, etc.

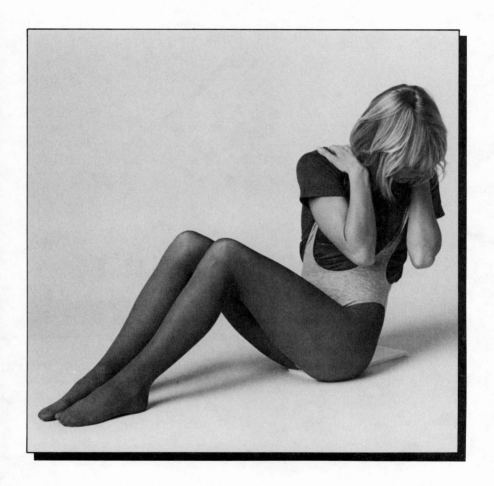

REVERSE LEG LIFTS

Assume a supine position and lift yourself up on your hands and heels. Extend your right leg forward with your toes pointed and slowly lift your right leg to hip level, then lower in succession. Repeat with your left leg. *Note:* Keep your back straight and your hips held up so your back does not sag.

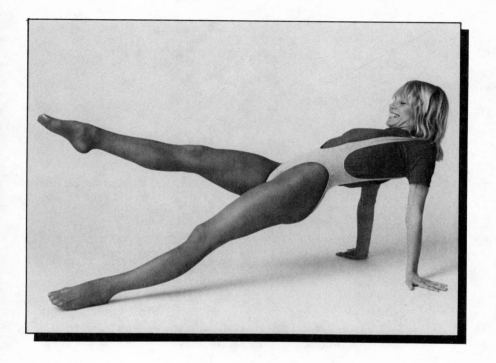

SEAT WALK

Sit with your knees bent and your arms held out level to your shoulders with your elbows slightly bent for balance. Bring your knees toward your chest and "scoot" along the floor by lifting and moving from one side of your buttocks to the other (keep your feet up off the floor). Use your arms and torso to increase your forward motion. Try to seat walk for several feet, then relax and repeat.

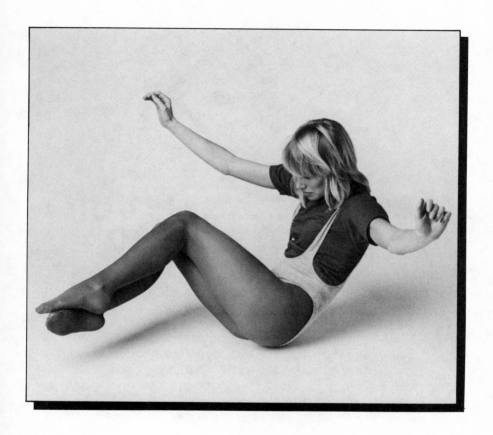

DOUBLE LEG LIFT UP AND OVERHEAD

Assume a supine position with your arms out at your shoulders. Bend your knees to your chest and extend both your legs up and over your head to touch the floor with your toes. Then slowly lift both your legs up toward the ceiling (with your toes pointed) and hold for 4-6 seconds. Return to the knee-chest position, and to the floor or starting position. Relax and repeat. *Note:* Do not support your lower back with your hands. Be sure that you are sufficiently "warmed-up" prior to performing this exercise.

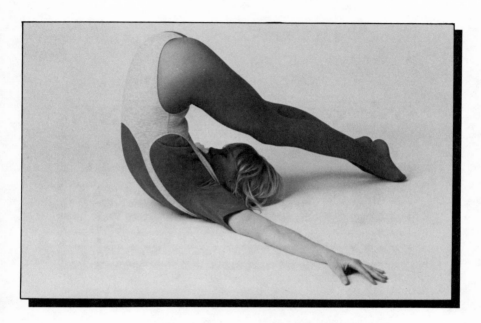

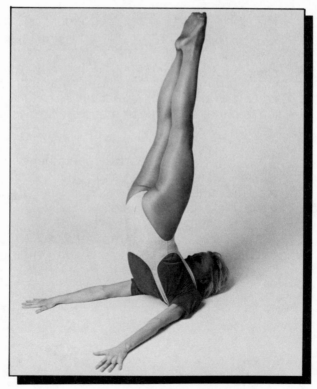

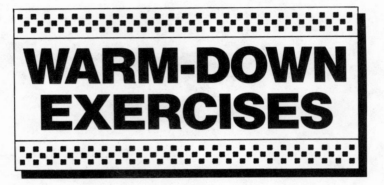

WARM-DOWN EXERCISES

After performing stomach exercises, you should do a few warm-down activities to prevent "pooling" of waste products in specific muscle groups. Appropriate activities should involve most of the larger muscle groups in your body and may include a warm bath or shower. There are many possible activities from which to choose. We recommend the following (at a minimum):

1 Walk around the room for a minutes, simultaneously doing a continuous series of exaggerated movements—step high, swing arms, shake legs, circle arms, circle head, etc.

2 Jump around loosely shaking out your arms and legs; alternate jumping on one foot, the other, and both feet.

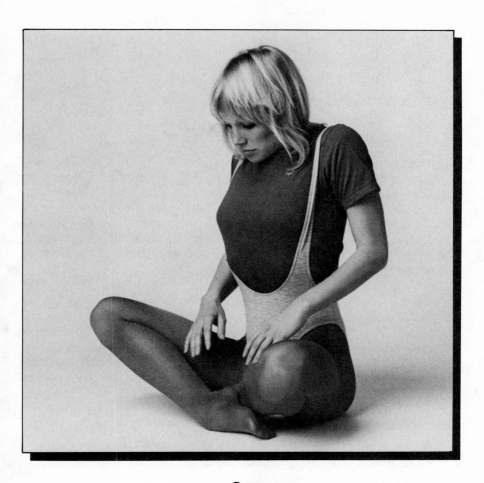

3 Repeat warm-up exercises #1 (head circles and shoulder shrugs) and #2 cross sitting stretches.

THE AUTHORS

Dr. James A. Peterson is the Director of Sports Medicine for the Women's Sports Foundation. The author of more than 20 books on sports and fitness, Dr. Peterson taught for over nine years at the United States Military Academy in West Point, New York. While on the faculty at West Point, he conducted several pioneer studies in the areas of strength training and the physical training of women. After West Point, he served as a fitness consultant to the Department of Athletics at Stanford University.

Susan L. Peterson is a free-lance writer who resides in Kensington, California. As the first woman instructor in the history of the United States Military Academy, she has appeared several times on national television, including the Johnny Carson Tonight Show. A fitness and self-defense expert, she has written several books and articles in national publications, including *People* magazine. The books she has authored include: *An Improved Figure Through Exercise, Self Defense for Women — The West Point Way, The Women's Stretching Book,* and *The Women's Self Defense Book — How to Stay Safe and Fight Back.*